# From Einkorn Wheat to GMO

# Other books by this author

- Microscopic Colitis
- Understanding Microscopic Colitis
- Vitamin D and Autoimmune Disease
- 8 Ways to Prevent Pancreatic Cancer

# From Einkorn Wheat to GMO

## A Quick Look at the Evolution of Genetics in Agricultural Crops

Wayne Persky

**Persky Farms**

United States

**First published and distributed in the United States of America by:**
Persky Farms, 19242 Darrs Creek Rd, Bartlett, TX 76511-4460. Tel.: (1)254-718-1125; Fax: (1)254-527-3682. www.perskyfarms.com



**Disclaimer and Legal Notice:** The information contained in this book is intended solely for general educational purposes, and is not intended, nor implied, to be a substitute for professional medical advice relative to any specific medical condition or question. The advice of a physician or other health care provider should always be sought for any questions regarding any medical condition. Specific diagnoses and therapies can only be provided by the reader's physician. Any use of the information in this book is at the reader's discretion. The author and the publisher specifically disclaim any and all liability arising directly or indirectly from the use or application of any information contained in this book.

Please note that much of the information in this book is based on personal experience and anecdotal evidence. Although the author and publisher have made every reasonable attempt to achieve complete accuracy of the content, they assume no responsibility for errors or omissions. If you should choose to use any of this information, use it according to your best judgment, and at your own risk. Because your particular situation will not exactly match the examples upon which this information is based, you should adjust your use of the information and recommendations to fit your own personal situation.

This book does not recommend or endorse any specific tests, products, procedures, opinions, or other information that may be mentioned anywhere in the book. This information is provided for educational purposes, and reliance on any tests, products, procedures, or opinions mentioned in the book is solely at the reader's own risk.

Any trademarks, service marks, product names, or named features are assumed to be the property of their respective owners, and are used only for reference. There is no implied endorsement when these terms are used in this book.



ISBN 978-1-7320792-5-0

# Contents

# Introduction

The author grew up on a small family farm in Central Texas during the 1940's and 50s. After the end of World War II in 1945, the world was recovering from all the destruction and the loss of so many lives, and agriculture in the United States was still recovering from the devastating drought of the 1930s. A lot of good farmers had no choice but to leave farming and go to work in factories or wherever they could find employment after so many years of poor crop production due to the extended drought.

Originally, agriculture had been a labor-intensive occupation and most of the labor involved long hours and back-breaking work. But improved mechanization was beginning to take the place of hand labor for certain chores, especially for harvesting operations.

But the increased productivity soon brought surpluses, and commodity prices steadily declined. Farmers had to increase their production, in order to make a living, so they used more fertilizer, and better and better hybrid corn seed, and they were indeed able to increase production. But that just drove prices even lower.

When most manufacturers realize that they are producing much more than the market needs, resulting in excessive inventory surpluses that are accompanied by depressed prices, they either reduce their production rate, or they find a way to decrease costs or increase demand for their products, in order to sustain profitability.

Farmers don't generally follow that pattern. Farmers are born to produce, and no matter how price-depressing the surpluses might be, farmers continue to produce more. They are continually adopting new ways to increase production and efficiency, because ultimately, increasing production is their passion.

But of course the first technological advances in agriculture did not occur in the 1940s. Agriculture first appeared on the planet roughly 10,000 years ago when grain production first became possible as a result of what was probably a natural accidental hybridization event. The cross-breeding of Einkorn wheat and a species of goat grass resulted in a form of hybrid wheat, known as emmer wheat. That lucky event was followed by a second hybrid crossing which gave neolithic people the first wheat variety that was capable of producing superior bread dough.

After that fortuitous beginning thousands of years ago, growers have since been able to coax many, ,many minor genetic innovations out of wheat in order to increase agricultural production potential over the millennia. But arguably the most substantial changes that have ever occurred in the history of the genetics of cereal grains happened with those two hybridizations, long, long ago. And they probably occurred by some act of nature, rather than as a result of human intervention.

If this book does nothing else, I sincerely hope that it will increase your understanding of crop genetics and how important the issue is in our lives, and in the continuing evolution of our species. I hope that it will help you to understand how we got to where we are and how we can sort out the food-related priorities of today so that we will continue to thrive not only as individuals, but as a species. In the game of life, our survival is always at stake, so our choices matter — a lot.

# Chapter 1

# In The Beginning, Life Was Good

## For at least a couple of million years, prehuman and human ancestors hunted and gathered their food in the abundance of nature.

When humans first began to develop the physical and mental characteristics that eventually distinguished their descendants as uniquely human, and as they developed the skills that would eventually drive them to the top of the food chain, agriculture did not exist. Paleoanthropologists tell us that according to the fossil records, modern humans (Homo sapiens) first appeared approximately 200,000 years ago. Wild game and edible plants were plentiful where Homo sapiens roamed. So early humans lived off the land by hunting wild game, catching fish, or gathering fruit, nuts, and seeds from trees and bushes, and by digging up tubers and roots of certain plants. Life was good.

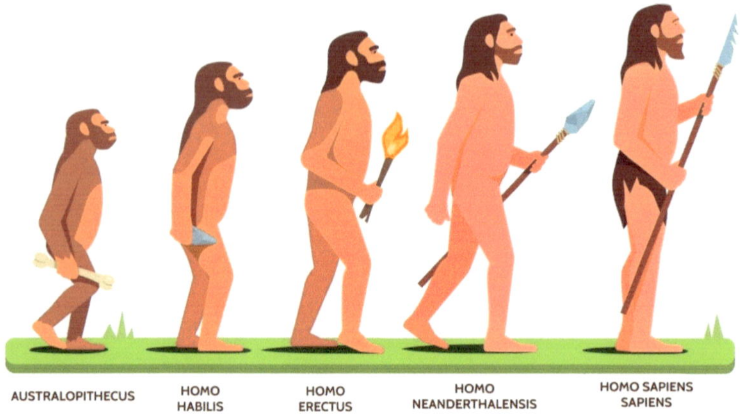


*Illustration 1: Artist's depiction of the evolution of humans (Homo sapiens).*

## And most importantly, life was simple.

Sure, there were occasional conflicts with other large predators or other tribes. And some years, and especially during certain seasons, adverse weather or other environmental conditions could cause animals and edible plants to become scarce. Fires caused by lightening strikes could wipe out huge areas of grassland and even forests, destroying most of the plants and driving the animals out. But when the rains came, within weeks new plants would begin to emerge and wild animals would return to graze on the fresh growth. Occasionally going to bed hungry was probably a common occurrence back in those days, but eventually, one way or another, nature always provided, and humans prospered.

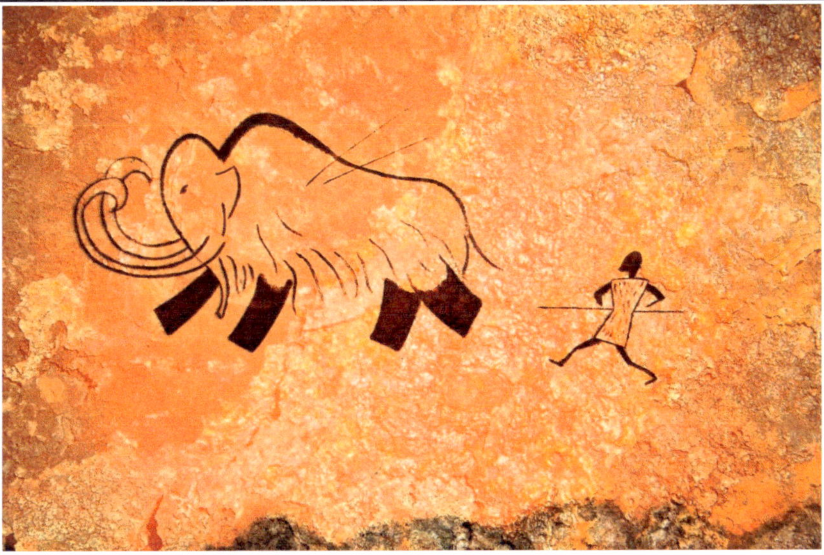

*Illustration 2: Cave art depicting a woolly mammoth hunt.*

## Fast forward to the neolithic period in the history of human evolution.

Life for the nomadic tribes of hunter-gatherers was becoming increasingly difficult. Not only were the once plentiful supplies of wild game animals and edible plants becoming more difficult to find with each passing season, but the competition for the remaining pockets of food was leading to more frequent and more violent confrontations with other tribes that also relied on the same sources of food. And migrating to other areas held little advantage, because eventually it became almost impossible to find territory that wasn't either already hunted out, with few edible plants and animals remaining, or the tribes that were already there were willing and able to defend their claim to that territory. Life was becoming tougher with each passing year.

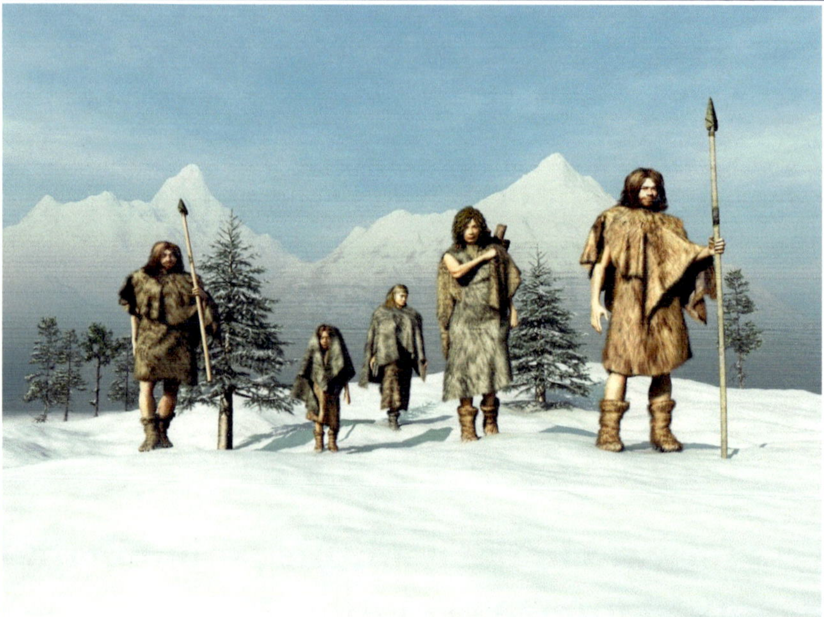

*Illustration 3: As the human population continued to grow, game animals and edible plants became increasingly difficult to find as humans searched for new territory.*

## But as the situation becomes increasingly desperate, wheat comes to the rescue.

The archaeological evidence suggests that humans living in the area of the Fertile Crescent in the Middle East had been gathering wild wheat seed for food for thousands of years before cultivation was ever attempted. By a stroke of good fortune (for neolithic period humans), wheat happens to be a rather genetically-unique species.

## Normally, cross-breeding of 2 different species yields offspring that are sterile.

This applies to plants, animals, and all other advanced forms of life. But somewhere between 10,000 and 40,000 years ago a wild wheat species, einkorn (Triticum monococcum), crossed with a species of goat grass (Aegilops speltoides) and produced fertile offspring.

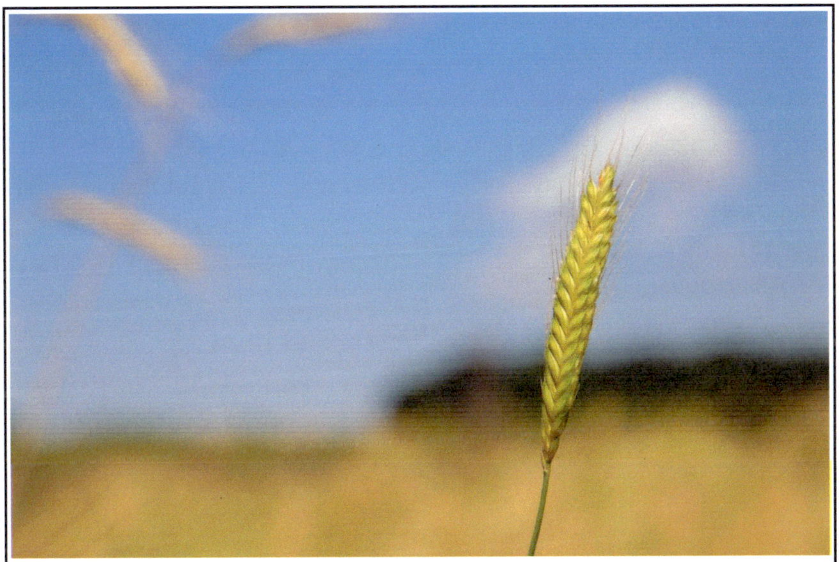

*Illustration 4: Einkorn wheat (Triticum monococcum).*

When botanists discuss wheat breeding, they often point out that wheat is more complex than other cereal grains. And they aren't exaggerating. Every cell of every living creature contains deoxyribonuceic acid ( DNA). And that DNA contains the instructions that define all the processes necessary for life and replication. DNA is structured as long ribbon-like strands known as chromosomes. Various species have evolved in various ways, so some have more chromosomes than others. And organisms tend to have differing numbers of copies of chromosomes.

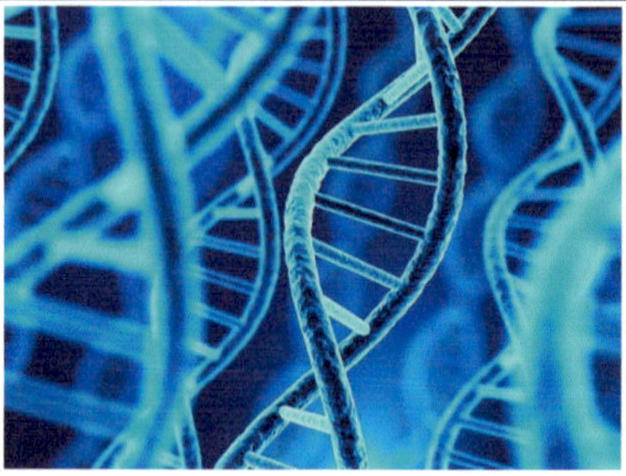

*Illustration 5: Deoxyribonucleic acid (DNA) is normally depicted as a double helix chain of nucleotides.*

For example a human cell has 23 pairs of chromosomes, for a total of 46 chromosomes. This is known as a diploid arrangement. By contrast, wheat cells have a hexaploid arrangement — six copies of its seven chromosomes for a total of 42 chromosomes. Corn has a total of 20 chromosomes and rice has a total of 24. Interestingly, wheat, corn, and rice are technically all grasses and they all originated from a common ancestor over 50 million years ago, but they have all evolved quite differently over the years.

Although wheat has fewer chromosomes than humans, it has many more genes. Wheat has somewhere between 164,000 and 334,000 genes, while humans have only 20,000 to 25,000 genes (Colorado wheat, 2013, Nov 15).[1]

The entire set of genetic material that contains the instructions for the reproduction and functioning of an organism is known as the genome of that organism. Among the commonly grown crops, wheat has the largest genome.

## Einkorn wheat is a diploid and has only 14 chromosomes.

But the result of that first fortuitous cross-breeding gave our ancestors wild emmer wheat, which is a tetraploid with 28 chromosomes (in comparison with the hexaploid arrangement of 42 chromosomes of modern wheat). As mentioned previously, this cross-breeding apparently occurred between two wild species, without human intervention.

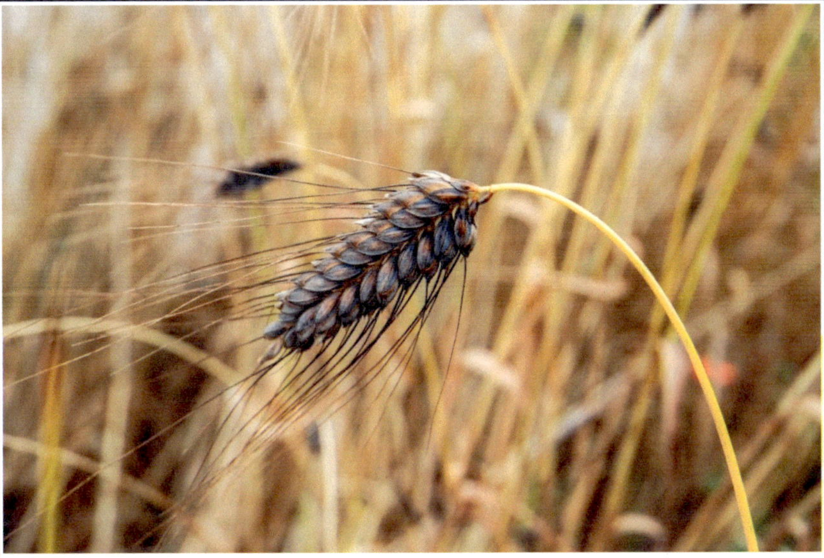

*Illustration 6: Emmer wheat (Triticum turgidum).*

## If the hybridization had resulted in a diploid (two sets of chromosomes), the offspring would have been sterile.

But the extra chromosomes in four sets of chromosomes allowed the cross to be fertile. The earliest clear evidence of the agricultural production of domesticated emmer wheat ranges from about 7,650 to 8,200 years BC near Damascus, Syria (Encyclopedia of life, n.d,).[2]

Einkorn wheat may have been domesticated sooner than emmer wheat. The earliest known production of einkorn wheat occurred in southeastern Turkey about 7,950 to 8,650 BC (Encyclopedia of life, n.d.).[3] But wild emmer wheat was gathered for thousands of years before this, so it's possible that it was grown as a crop elsewhere earlier than einkorn wheat.

## The second lucky cross-breeding took place about 7,000 BC.

Wild emmer (known as Triticum turgidum subspecies dicoccoides) and another species of goat grass (Aegilops tauschii) crossed to yield Triticum aestivum, which is a hexaploid with 42 chromosomes (Crop Origins, n.d.).[4] It has become the basis for modern wheat and it has led to the development of over 25,000 (by some estimates) cultivars of bread wheat since then (Encyclopedia of life, n.d.).[5]

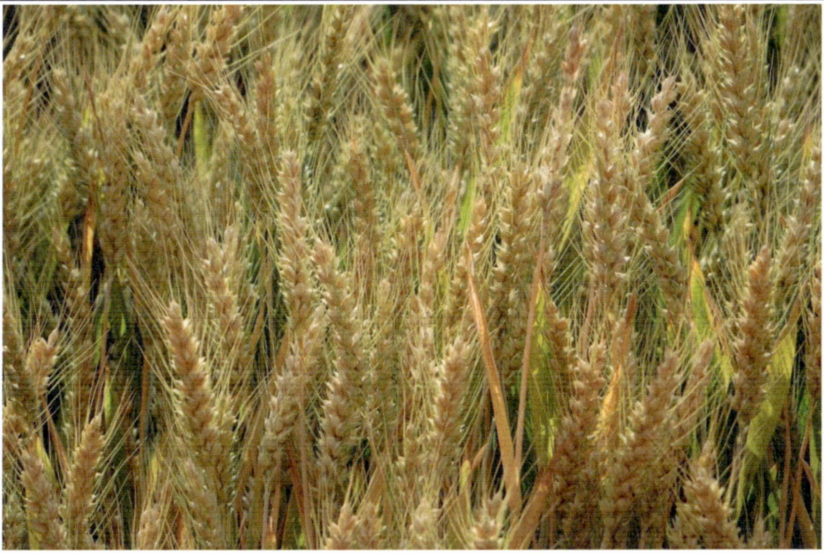

*Illustration 7: Common bread wheat (Triticum aestivm).*

The seed pods of wild plants tend to shatter in order to scatter the seeds. As cereal grain plants are domesticated, they are selected for tighter husks which will help to hold the seeds tighter and longer to reduce loses before harvest. Over the years farmers select plants with more and larger grain, to further enhance yields. But the main benefit of the emmer/goat grass cross was the addition of 2 or 3 genes that upgraded the proteins that create elasticity in the dough when kneaded. This upgrade in the quality of the gluten in wheat was what makes wheat so uniquely suited for bread-making.

**But note that this hybridization resulted in a plant that produced grain that had a new molecular structure in some of it's proteins.** Humans had not evolved with these proteins. Consequently, they could not completely digest some of the proteins in wheat. Normally, digestion results in breaking down the molecules in food into individual amino acids so that they can be used by the body as building blocks for new tissue. But digestion of wheat results in incomplete digestion. Molecules are composed of long strings of amino acids, and the human digestive system is not capable of completely cleaving parts of the gluten molecules in wheat. This results in certain short and medium-length chains of amino acids (known as peptides). These peptides provoke increased intestinal permeability (leaky gut) and they manage to escape the digestive system and get into the bloodstream of anyone who is sensitive to wheat gluten. They are the apparent cause of celiac disease.

Some wanna-be authorities claim that advancements in wheat breeding methods to increase gluten content in wheat that were made roughly half a century ago are the main cause of a recent perception that gluten sensitivity is increasing. That's simply not true. The major changes in wheat genetics were made in that second prehistoric hybridization when bread wheat (Triticum aestivum) was created by the cross-breeding of emmer wheat and a species of goat grass (Aegilops tauschii). Every modification in the wheat genome that has been made since that second hybridization event can only be described as part of a series of comparatively minor refinements, whether the changes have occurred as a result of natural selection, or genetically modified organism (GMO) technology. The increase in celiac diagnoses that has occurred since then is due more to increased awareness of celiac disease, than to any changes in wheat seed breeding. As physicians become more aware of a medical condition they are more likely to look for it in their patients, and this naturally boosts the diagnostic rate.

## It's the gluten in wheat that causes celiac disease.

Gluten is primarily made up of two protein fractions, namely prolamins (storage proteins) and glutelins. All grains contain a form of gluten, but only the gluten in wheat, rye, and barley have been pinpointed as triggers for celiac disease.

The prolamins in wheat are called gliadins and the glutelins are known as glutenins. Both of these protein fractions have been shown to cause adverse reactions in people who are sensitive to them. And as mentioned above most people who are sensitive to the gluten components in wheat are also sensitive to the prolamins in rye (known as secalin) and barley (known as hordein). In addition, many of those same individuals are sensitive to the prolamin (known as avenin) in oats. Rice is the only other grain for which a glutelin is commonly mentioned (orycenin), but very rarely are people sensitive to it, and it is not associated with celiac disease.

Wheat digestion results in many different gliadin and glutenin peptides to which celiacs are known to react, but the digestion of rye, barley, or oats produces far fewer reactive peptides. Altogether, this group of grains has been shown to be associated with hundreds of different peptides that can provoke immune system responses (from people who are sensitive to them) (Tye-Din et al., 2010).[6]

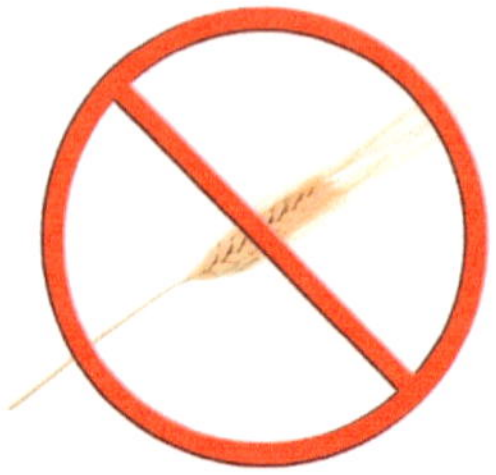

*Illustration 8: Celiac disease is caused by certain proteins found in gluten in wheat.*

A description of celiac disease can be found in the medical literature of approximately 2,000 years ago (Guandalini, 2007, summer. p. 1).[7] But until the 1920s, the medical community was clueless as to what caused celiac disease, so they had no idea how to treat it. Considering that celiac disease is a relatively simple disease caused by a sensitivity to gluten, with a straightforward treatment (avoid gluten), why has it taken the medical community almost 2,000 years to begin to address it? And after about another hundred years, why is their overall understanding of the disease still rather rudimentary? Some sources estimate that the diagnostic criteria are so primitive that as few as 5 % of all celiacs are ever even diagnosed. How could this be?

## The likely reason for this problem is due to inadequate training of physicians.

Traditionally, physicians have received very little (if any) training in diet and nutrition. They're taught to diagnose health problems and treat them either by surgery or by prescribing a drug-based treatment. Consequently they are unable to even intelligently consider the issues caused by food sensitivities in their patients. Even though food sensitivities are at the root of many modern health problems, physicians are generally unable to even recognize the association, let alone understand how to properly treat food sensitivities.

## Most doctors simply don't understand food sensitivities.

And they don't understand the differences between food allergies, food sensitivities, and other gastrointestinal issues well enough to be able to tell the difference. This was well illustrated by a study sponsored by several regulatory agencies of the U. S. government, as well as a number of industry organizations focused on food allergies (National Academies of Sciences et al., 2017).[8] The study clearly showed that most medical professionals don't understand these issues and aren't equipped to treat them. They don't even have adequate testing methods available to them.

And part of the blame may be attributed to the excessive reliance of many physicians on their drug reps. Far too many physicians rely on their drug reps from the pharmaceutical companies to provide them with continued education in the form of up-to-date information on treatment methods. The drug reps can hardly be blamed for omitting information and training on any issue that does not require drugs as part of the treatment. It shouldn't be surprising that physicians don't understand gluten sensitivity very well, and that they often tend to overlook it, in view of the fact that it is so deemphasized in their continuing education.

# Chapter 2

# Our Ancestors Ate a Simple Diet for Millions of Years

## Originally, humans were primarily meat-eaters.

The claim that our paleo ancestors ate a lot of carbohydrates as part of their normal diet is an illusion promoted by health advocates who misinterpret the archaeological evidence. It's unclear whether they misinterpret the evidence intentionally (in order to promote their agenda) or innocently (because of a lack of scientific sophistication) , but as a result, much of the widely-published information about paleolithic diets overemphasizes the amount of carbohydrates and fiber in typical paleolithic diets.

## Early humans and their ancestors were meat-eaters.

Yes, paleolithic period humans ate carbohydrates sometimes, especially if they needed to keep from starving when they couldn't acquire enough meat. And they apparently ate berries and various fruit when it was in season, but this only happened during relatively limited times of the year. As a rule, carbohydrates were generally a relatively minor part of their diet. Our competitive success as a species was due to the fact that we evolved eating mainly meat (Wanjek, 2012, Nov 26; Choi, 2012, Oct 3, Choi, (2011, Dec 13).[9, 10, 11]

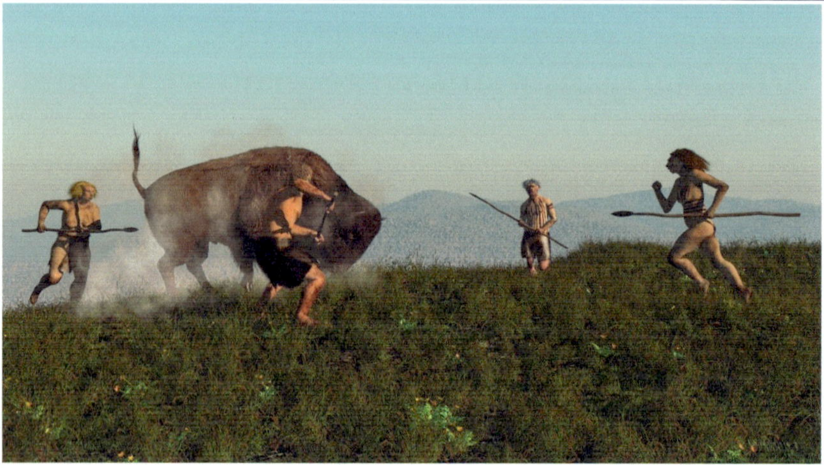

*Illustration 9: Stone age bison hunters.*

Consider the fact that gorillas are roughly three times the size of humans, but they have evolved with smaller brains. How could that be? The dramatic difference almost surely has to be due to their traditional vegan diet, which is devoid of any animal-based protein.

But the clearest evidence that humans evolved as meat-eaters has come from Scandinavia where osteologists recently examined the bones of people who lived in southern Scandinavia during the period from about 10,500 years ago to 7,500 years ago (Lund University, 2018, Mar 19).[12] They found that at one settlement, slightly over 50 % of the diet came from fish, 10 % came from seals, 37 % came from land animals such as deer and wild boar, and only about 3 % came from plants such as berries, nuts, and mushrooms.

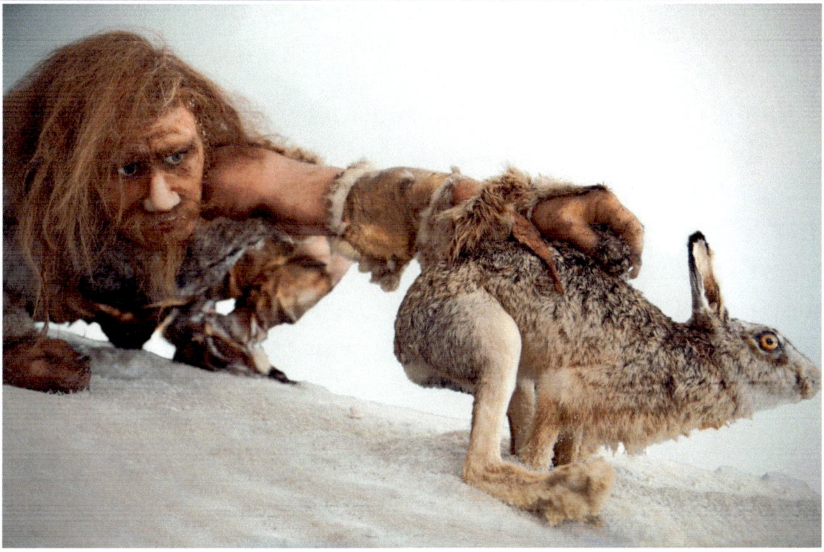

*Illustration 10: Caveman catching a hare.*

On a nearby island where there were no land animals other than hares, almost 60 % of the ingested protein came from fish and almost 40 % of the protein came from seals. Hares and vegetables were a negligible part of the diet.

## Big brains consume more energy.

Most people assume that energy expenditure equates to the use of muscles. You might be surprised to learn that when at rest, your brain consumes about 20 % of your body's energy uses, about twice the amount of the brains of other primates. It takes a significant amount of energy to keep a big brain functioning properly and nutritionists and dietitians seem to have lost sight of that fact today.

Although meat was the preferred fuel for humans during the paleolithic period, when facing starvation, most people will eat almost anything in order to survive. And that was the situation that led to the neolithic period of our evolution. Population growth had resulted in over-hunting, and the result was an acute shortage of meat sources. The decision to settle down and develop agriculture was seen as a way to prevent mass starvation.

The second reference cited on a previous page (back two pages) describes the examination of the remains of a prehuman infant who had died about 1.5 million year ago (Choi, 2012, October 3). The cause of death was apparently malnutrition. An examination of the pieces of skull showed that the child had porotic hyperostosis, which is a type of spongy bone growth caused by insufficient availability of dietary iron, folate, and vitamin B-12. That particular condition is due to a deficiency of animal-based products in the diet of a species that requires them. Plants cannot provide B-12 —B-12 is only available in animal-based products. And B12 is essential for brain development.

The child was about old enough for weaning. Either the mother was unable to supply breast milk that contained the essential nutrients, or the child's diet did not contain adequate animal products. Regardless of the reason, this is evidence that meat had to be a regular (not just occasional) part of the prehuman diet at least a million or more years ago. Where humans evolved on the African savanna, meat was plentiful.

This is not to say that vegan and vegetarian diets cannot be beneficial for health. They can be, especially in certain situations. But according to our evolutionary history, they should not be considered natural, because they were not a primary part of our evolutionary diet. They were mainly invoked as a maintenance ration during periods when meat supplies were inadequate.

## The neolithic period in our history brought dramatic lifestyle changes.

When humans were forced to embrace agricultural development during the neolithic period in order to prevent starvation, the dietary shock had to present some major problems. The transition from eating a primarily meat-based diet to eating a primarily plant-based diet resulted in a deficiency of protein and fat, and initiated a long decline in the general health of the human species. Today, approximately 300 generations later, we continue to show the signs of continuing deterioration of the general health of our species. Obviously, feeding a population of carnivores a plant-based diet and expecting them to thrive is unrealistic at best, and ludicrous at worst.

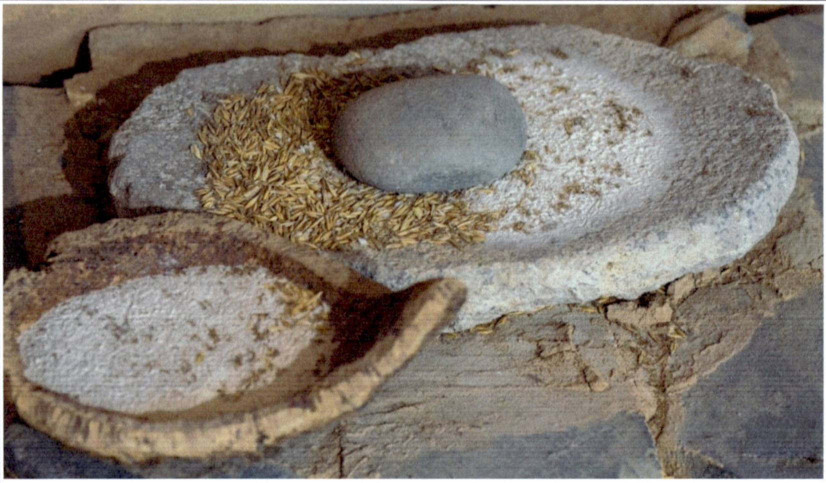

*Illustration 11: Neolithic tools for grinding grain.*

Jared Diamond pointed out this dilemma rather eloquently in 1987 when he wrote an article (which became famous) for Discover Magazine in which he described agriculture as "*The Worst Mistake in the History of the Human Race*" (Diamond, 1987, May).[13] In that article he pointed out (among other things) that the hunter-gatherers who lived prior to the neolithic period were generally healthier, taller, lived longer, had less disease, had more leisure time, and various other virtues, compared with their neolithic descendants. And in the next-to-last paragraph, he described the reason why this mistake was made and why the decision to develop agriculture was inevitable.(Diamond, 1987, May)

> *At this point it's instructive to recall the common complaint that archaeology is a luxury, concerned with the remote past, and offering no lessons for the present. Archaeologists*

> *studying the rise of farming have reconstructed a crucial stage at which we made the worst mistake in human history. Forced to choose between limiting population or trying to increase food production, we chose the latter and ended up with starvation, warfare, and tyranny.*(pp. 64–66)

Perhaps the most striking observation about Diamond's article is that while he listed wheat and other cereal grains, he didn't even mention the addition of gluten to the human diet. Therefore he didn't even consider the consequences to the human digestive system brought on by adding wheat to the diet. Instead he chose to view the issue as a general decline in human health caused not just by wheat, but by the shift to agriculturally-produced food in general. It could certainly be argued that wheat gluten was the primary cause for the decline in human health, although it's true that dairy products, soy, and other cereal grains have caused significant damage to human health, also. At any rate, Diamond's article generally condemned agriculture, rather than criticizing any specific part of it.

## Was the Bible possibly the first book to disparage agriculture?

In Genesis, Adam and Eve are described as living in paradise. After they were disobedient, Adam's punishment was to be required to farm (a hard, sweaty job). Apparently, the connotation was that farm life was not a desirable way of life. Whether this was the actual intent or not, the agricultural "revolution" has resulted in us being able to produce more food per person, even surpluses, but at what cost? These days the healthcare system seems to focus on the challenges of keeping fatter, less healthy people alive longer.

Humans can certainly subsist on a vegan diet, or some version of the modern Western diet of today. But we would have never been able to develop our relatively big brains and rise to the top of the food chain if we had been restricted to those kinds of diets during our evolution.

Without a meat-based diet during our development, we would be just another primate species today, provided that we would have been able to compete well enough to maintain territorial rights on this planet. It's more likely that we wouldn't have been able to compete with other species, and we wouldn't have survived as a species. After all, out of all the species that have ever lived on this planet, approximately 99 % are now extinct.

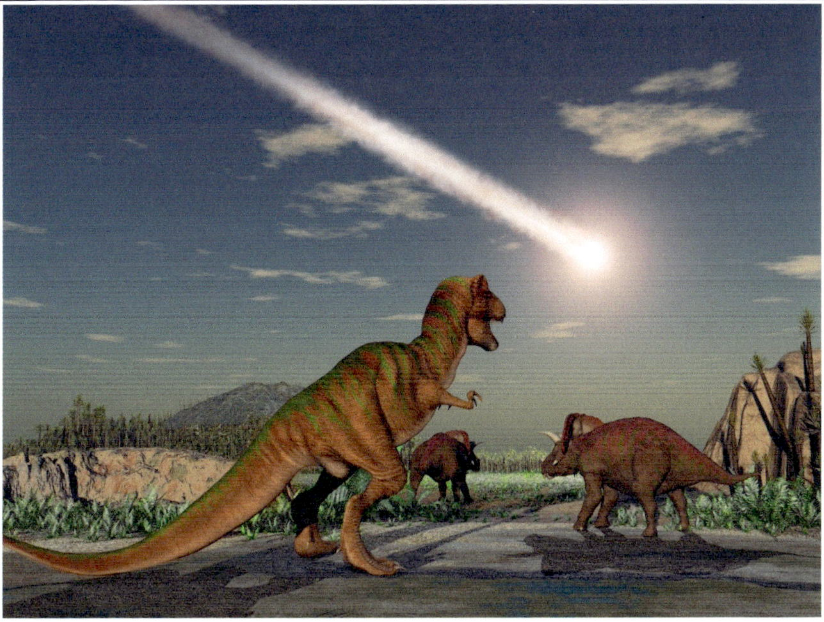

*Illustration 12: Artist's rendition of the asteroid event known as Chicxulub that caused the sudden mass extinction of the dinosaurs and about three-quarters of the plant and animal species that existed on earth at the time, approximately 66 million years ago.*

# Chapter 3

# Why the GMO Issue Should Remind Us of Déjà Vu

## Revolt against technological advances in agriculture has been surprisingly common throughout history.

If we review the history of agriculture, it's not an all surprising that GMO technology would inspire protests and resentment. There are no apparent records of how well neolithic humans accepted the adoption of those early wheat crosses that enabled farming as a practical venture, but it would probably be safe to guess that they were met with more than slight skepticism. Throughout history, agricultural innovations have almost always met with opposition.

When a Berkshire farmer invented a crude grain drill in 1701 to simplify and speed up the planting of small gains such as wheat, it brought an outcry of resentment. When a threshing machine was developed about a century later, it was met with riots.

**From Einkorn Wheat to GMO**

In the early part of the 1900's, when the process for making ammonia by combining nitrogen from the air with hydrogen from coal was discovered, the prospect of using nitrogen fertilizer instead of manure was about as appealing to many farmers as the plague. Similar to the perception behind fears of GMO technology, the impression was that synthetic fertilizer wasn't natural like manure, so it couldn't be acceptable. So the new technology saw limited use for many years.

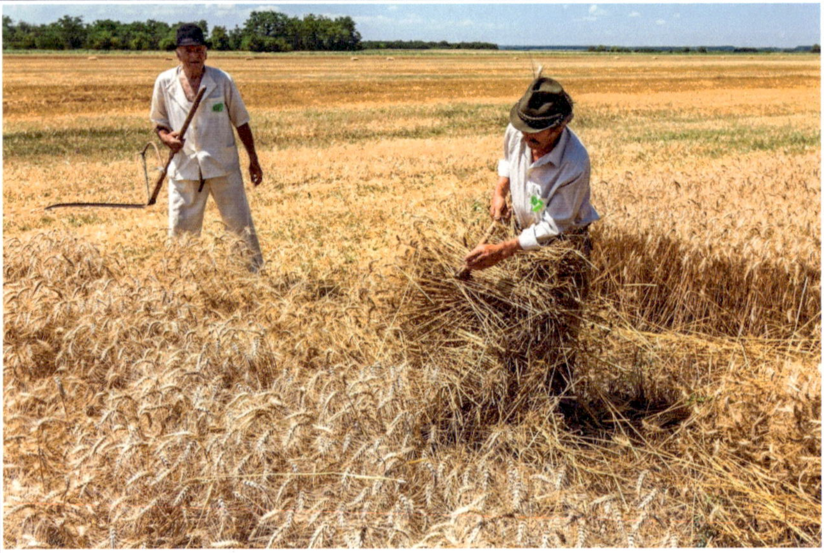

*Illustration 13: Harvesting wheat with hand tools prior to the development of machines to do the work*

For thousands of years, farming required so much manual labor that many workers were needed in order to produce relatively small amounts of grain (compared with today's production methods). Consequently, most people were farmers. But when industrialization came along, many people moved into the cities and became factory workers. This created an extra push for the development of machinery that could replace human labor on the farm.

## When most people were farmers, the opinions of farmers really mattered.

By about 1850, the number of farmers was down to about 64 % of the working population (at least in the U.S.), and by 1920, it was down to about 30 %.[14] Today less than 2 % of the population are farmers. And many of these are not full-time farmers, so they do not actually earn their living as farmers. The number of full-time farmers is less than 1 %.[15] So the fact that farmers seem to be embracing GM technology hardly affects the overall perception of it because the bulk of the population sees it as a threat.

## Historically, the DNA of cereal grains has been altered by x-rays, thermal neurons, and harsh chemicals.

Interestingly, for decades modern cereal grain scientists have been using x-rays, thermal neurons, and harsh chemicals such as ethyl methanesulphonate to damage the DNA and produce mutations in cereal grains. In fact, most of the wheat and barley varieties being grown today were produced by mutations of this sort. There were no safety tests done, and no one protested.

In 1983 the technique of using genetic modification (GM) was developed as a gentler, safer, more predictable alternative to breeding by mutations. Instead of selecting plants from a profusion of randomly generated mutations, agronomists could simply use GM to add the traits they desired. Not surprisingly, all hell broke loose.

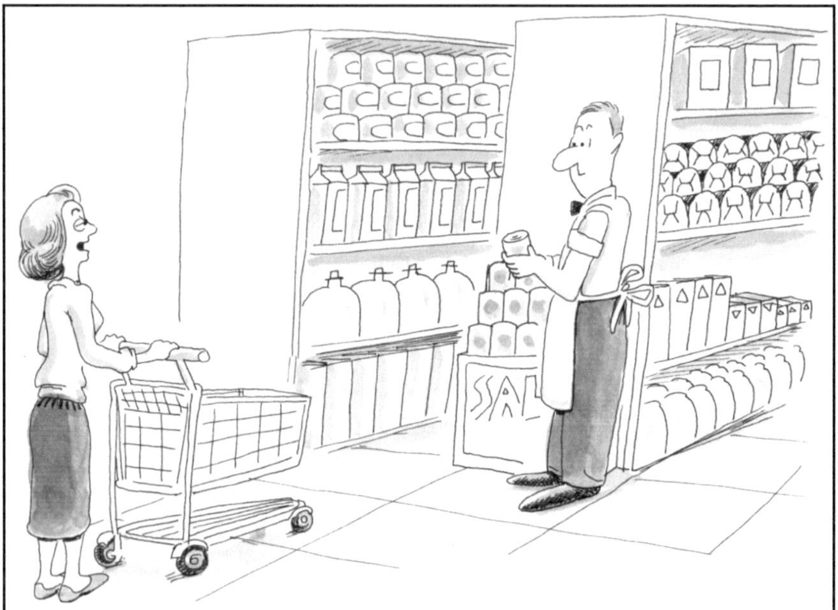

"In what aisle are the 'won't immediately kill you' foods?"

## To ensure that we're all on the same page as far as the discussions in this book are concerned, here is my definition of genetically modified organisms (GMOs).

**GMOs are living organisms in which certain genetic material has been manipulated artificially in a laboratory using genetic engineering techniques in order to specifically bestow a trait that was not previously present.** Usually, it involves a combination of plant, animal, bacteria, and virus genes to confer changes in properties that would not be likely to occur by means of traditional cross-breeding methods or by natural evolution. This should be a broad enough definition to satisfy most of us.

Does it seem strange that no one voiced any objections when modifications to plant genetics were based on random mutations caused by abusing genetic material, but as soon as scientists began to use an intelligent and orderly technique, the protests promptly surfaced? It's almost as if genetic manipulation by any sort of random methods, no matter how harsh, are fine — but as soon as we begin to make those changes in an orderly, intelligent fashion, the procedure is no longer acceptable.

Why should that be the case? Why would genetic manipulation by random methods be acceptable, while changes made by intelligent methods are not? Do we subconsciously view this as "playing God"? But according to an article by Philip Ball, the phrase "playing God" is a meaningless and dangerous cliché.[16]

Ball's article, incidentally, was inspired by an accomplishment of Craig Venter, who had recently made the headlines when he created the first artificial life form. Venter created a micro-organism with an entirely synthetic, designed genome. It was the first organism since life began on earth that is capable of reproducing, and that has a genome that is not derived primarily from one or more parent organisms.

And Ball reminds us of the quote by the British geneticist and evolutionary biologist John Burdon Sanderson Haldane, who said, "There is no great invention, from fire to flying, which has not been hailed as an insult to some god." So evidently this attitude "comes with the turf", so to speak. Perhaps it's a quirk of human nature, or an evolutionary phenomenon. Maybe it's a reflection of the natural tendency for humans to fear the unknown. Whatever the reason, it apparently has been a common thread throughout recorded history, so it was probably a human trait long before then.

## We inherit almost all of our genes (DNA) from our parents.

This is known as vertical gene transfer. But not all of our genes come from our parents. We also have approximately 150 genes that our ancestors received from viruses as our species was evolving. This is known as horizontal gene transfer. Other organisms also contain horizontally-transferred genes from various organisms. So horizontal gene transfer is not unheard of in nature.

## GM methods are also horizontal gene transfers.

Basically, GM technology is applied to seeds used for agricultural production as follows (Technology Spotlight. (2017, Feb 1):[17]

*How GM seeds are developed:*

1. *The desired trait (like disease resistance or drought tolerance) is identified in nature.*
2. *The gene for the trait is transferred into the plant seed.*
3. *The plant is tested to ensure that it is safe for people, animals, and the environment.*
4. *After years of testing and approvals from governments around the world, the new seeds are available to farmers.*

Thanks to GM technology, maize (corn) and rice have seen major innovations. But despite unfounded claims to the contrary by some anti-GMO activists, wheat has largely been passed by in the GM revolution, presumably because of wheat's relatively complex, hexaploid genome. Relatively few GM varieties of wheat have been made available, and compared with the other cereal grains, those have only minor GM-based innovations.

## In 2016, the results of a survey about food and health issues were published.

The survey results show that Americans are changing their minds about what they consider to be healthful foods (Raymond, and Kubitz, 2016, May 11).[18] And apparently, rather than this change in attitude being inspired by personal insight, it appears as though the trend might be fueled (at least to some extent) by media influence.

Articles disparaging enriched refined grains, saturated fat, added sugars, and low-calorie sweeteners have been popular during recent years. Along with articles promoting whole grains, protein from plant sources, and natural sugars.

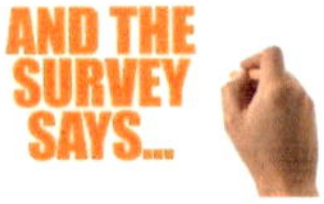


More and more Americans are choosing foods based on what they don't contain, rather than what they do contain. When asked to describe "healthful" foods (based on a list), over 40 % of respondents specifically mentioned "limited to no artificial ingredients or preservatives".

However, note that when it comes down to the nitty-gritty (when not prompted by a list), only about 2 % of consumers considered "limited or no artificial ingredients or preservatives" as a top consideration when selecting food. This wide variation in responses raises some serious questions about the validity of the conclusions stated for surveys of this type. Do conclusions based on such surveys really describe consumer trends, or do they merely reflect the goals of the investigators?

Looking at additional survey results, consumers are more likely to trust locally-produced food. While over 70% of respondents trust the safety of the food produced in their country, only 24 % trust the safety of food from other countries.

Not surprisingly, 70 % of Americans trust the food and food safety recommendations of registered dietitians or nutritionists. On the other hand, while 52 % (up from 42 % the year before) of Americans trust the food safety information issued by various United States government agencies, only 37 % get their diet recommendations from government agencies.

According to the survey results, Americans' food purchasing decisions are based on taste (84 %), price (71 %) perceived healthfulness (64 %), convenience (52%), and "sustainability" (41 %). 70 % of consumers believe that modern agriculture has at least some responsibility in providing a healthful food supply for everyone. 56 % believe that the food produced by modern agriculture is nutritious, and 53 % believe that it is safe.

73 % of the survey respondents support sustainability. However, note that only 38 % are willing to pay more for food that is produced by sustainable methods. Again, this probably reflects the agendas of the investigators and how the questions in the survey were phrased. In other words, if it doesn't cost them anything then sure, most consumers are in favor of sustainable farming methods But where the rubber meets the road, it's a different situation. Most Americans apparently believe that access to cheap, abundant, nutritious food is their birthright.

# Chapter 4

# Current Opinions

## Whose opinion is correct?

Between 1944 and 1963, while working with The Cooperative Wheat Research Production Program, Norman Borlaug managed to increase Mexico's wheat production by a factor of six (Nature Education, 2014).[19] He did this by using conventional selective breeding and cross-breeding techniques in order to reduce crop loses to the fungus known as stem rust.

Then he achieved similar spectacular results in other countries where there were food supply problems (including India and Pakistan). He initiated what has become known as the Green Revolution, and Norman Borlaug's contributions to crop production won him a Nobel Peace Prize in 1970.

Genetic modification entered the scene and began to take over crop breeding methods during the next few decades. The technology has allowed farmers to do things that were previously impossible, such as produce good yields of certain crops in hostile environments.

# Has GM technology actually brought increased food production?

Despite it's initial promise, in general, crop production increases that can be attributed to the use of GM technology appear to be no better than the previous yield trend that was established and maintained by selective breeding techniques. And now that public anti-GMO sentiment has reached the level where it is influencing governmental decisions, some countries have banned GM research and the production of GM crops.

It appears that approximately 70 % of packaged food contains some amount of GMO ingredients (The Times Editorial Board, 2016, May 21).[20] But as pointed out by that Los Angeles Times article, agronomists have been modifying the genetics of plants by cross-breeding and selective breeding for as long as we have been planting them and there have been no catastrophes so far. Without that genetic manipulation, many items in the produce sections of grocery stores would be difficult to recognize (in their original form).

Initially, the distinctions between conventional plant-breeding techniques and genetic engineering methods were obvious. But according to a report released in 2016 by the National Academies of Sciences, Engineering, and Medicine, those distinctions are no longer as clear.[21]

As an example to elucidate that claim, consider the genome editing technique known as CRISPR-Cas9. [22] CRISPR-Cas9, stands for clustered regularly interspaced short palindromic repeats and CRISPR-associated protein 9. Cas9 is an ribonucleic acid (RNA)-guided DNA endonuclease enzyme produced by the adaptive immune system of certain bacteria, such as Streptococcus pyogenes and others. The enzyme can be used as if it were a pair of "molecular scissors" to cut DNA strands at a specific location so that bits of DNA can then be added or removed.

## This idea was inspired by a technique that certain bacteria use to defend against attacks by viruses.

When a virus invades, the bacteria capture DNA snippets from the virus. They use the snippets to create segments known as CRISPR arrays which will provide a record that the bacteria can use in the future to identify the viruses (or similar viruses).

If at some point the bacteria detect a subsequent viral attack, they produce RNA segments from the CRISPR arrays to identify the virus. Then they use Cas9 (or a similar enzyme) to disable the virus by breaking down it's DNA. It's a very elegant and effective technique.

Scientists can use a similar process in the laboratory. They can create an RNA sequence that binds to the specific DNA that they wish to target. The RNA will also bind to the Cas9 enzyme and the Cas9 (or a similar enzyme) will cut the DNA at the desired location. The built-in repair abilities of the cell itself can then be used to add, delete, or replace a section of DNA with a customized sequence.

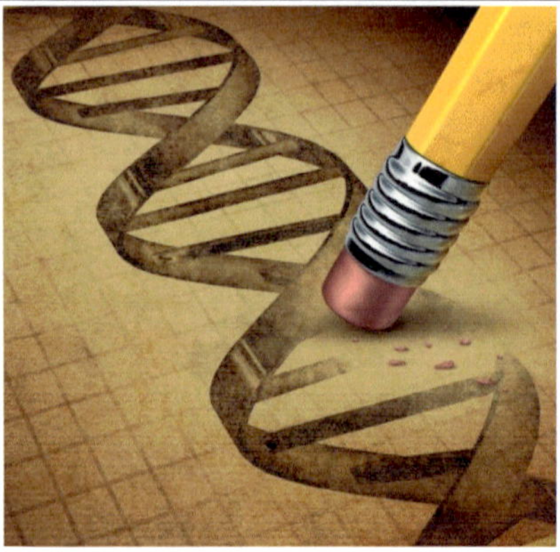

*Illustration 14: Scientists can remove, replace, or add material to a DNA segment.*

Scientists can either use this technique to splice DNA directly, or they can make the same genetic change by using radiation or chemicals to force the gene to mutate and then select the offspring with the desired mutation by using genetic screening. The result is the same. Since most authorities consider the latter process (using radiation or chemicals) to be a conventional plant breeding technique, we can begin to see how the previous distinctions between GM techniques and natural plant-breeding methods are fading away.

## The report highlighted some interesting observations.

For example, despite the fact that biologists have been able to use genetic engineering to produce characteristics such as longer shelf life, resistance to diseases, and higher vitamin content, the only GM characteristics that have been widely used commercially are those that allow a crop to tolerate certain herbicides and those that make a plant toxic to certain insect pests.

## Now why do you suppose that happened?

Probably it happened because the marketplace recognizes that farmers have demonstrated that they are willing to embrace GM and they are willing to pay for the technology, while consumers have demonstrated that they are not (not regarding food, anyway). Farmers will gladly pay for technology that gives them a production edge.

## Most consumers, on the other hand, tend to reject GM technology.

So they are certainly opposed to paying for it. While consumers say that they would like to have more nutritious, better-tasting food, they are not as willing to pay extra for it. Together with general consumer resistance toward GM-associated foods simply because of the GMO "stigma", this gives manufacturers and processors a relatively clear message that they are going to have a much tougher time trying to sell the idea to consumers. So while farmers have benefited from GM technology, the benefits to consumers have been more elusive.

## Farmers are eager to adopt new technology when they believe that it will make their work easier or increase their profit.

It seems somehow strangely ironic that farming is typically viewed by the general population as an occupation that requires, let's just say, less academic astuteness than most other careers. And yet farmers today tend to be very knowledgeable and they are early-adopters — eager to try new technology when it becomes available, provided that it shows promise for making their work more efficient or more profitable. Today, farming requires a good working knowledge of many, many technologies that were only a dream a generation ago. Imagine what farming might be like a generation from now into the future.

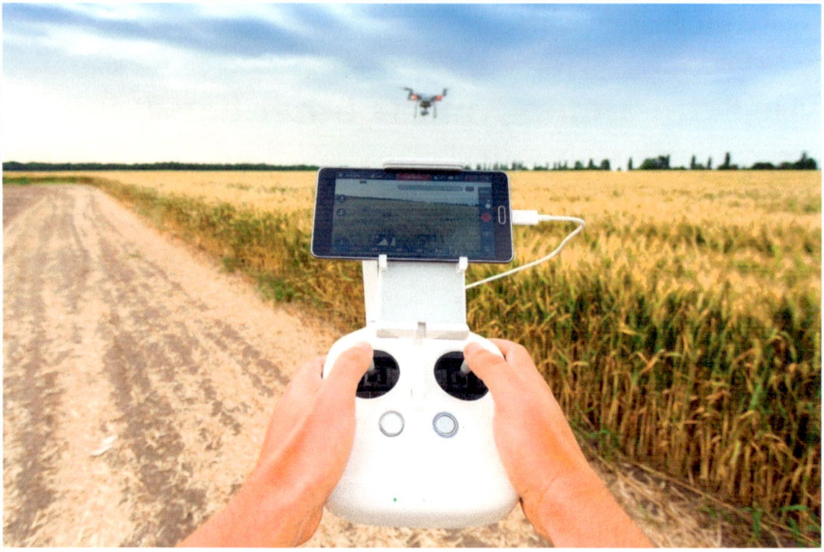

*Illustration 15: Checking a field with a drone*

Embracing the use of drones to check field and crop conditions, using GPS for automatic guidance of tractors and other machines, using electronics for automatic data collection and analysis, and accepting GMO are only a few examples of the uses of technology by farmers. Those who practice so-called "hobby farming" (part-time farming, or "weekend" farming) can certainly afford to ignore the latest technology. But farming is so competitive in today's world that full-time farmers can ill afford to use anything less than the latest technology if they hope to survive (or prosper). That means taking advantage of the benefits that GM technology has to offer concerning their chosen crop mix.

According to the United Nations, the world's population is expected to increase from about 7 billion to more than 9 billion people by 2050 (debating europe, n.d.).[23] They claim that global food production will need to be doubled by then in order to keep up with demand. And this must be done despite the fact that the amount of available farm land continues to shrink. Biotechnology may be the only way to meet that demand and provide enough food from less land.

## But as we've already noted, GM methods have not affected yield trends.

Interestingly, the National Academies of Sciences, Engineering, and Medicine report confirms that no change in the long-term rate of increase in crop production trends could be attributed to the use of GM. No evidence of a spike in production can be found. The long-term production trend continues to rise of course, but the rate of increase seems to be unchanged. So the claims by some proponents (including the United Nations) that GM technology is the only way to meet future food demands, are obviously not substantiated by this report.

And while some effect on human health,or changes to the environment might eventually become evident at some point in the future, the report found that so far at least, no adverse consequences can be attributed to the use of GM technology. There have been subtle changes, such as certain herbicide-resistant weeds, and insect-resistant plants that have lost some of their insect resistance, but when a program using GM technology is properly carried out, those risks are minimized. Naturally occurring adverse phenomena have been much more harmful to local environments over the years. Events such as the accidental introduction of the imported fire ant and killer bees, zebra mussels, giant salvinia and other invasive plants in the southern U. S. tend to be much greater threats.

## And then of course there is the pretty-much opposite opinion shared by anti-GMO advocates.

During the past decade or so, countless blogs have appeared on the Internet describing various reasons why GM technology is inherently dangerous for humans and most of the creatures and plants that inhabit this planet. After reading some of those blogs, one can't help but wonder why we haven't already become extinct (after all, this has been going on for decades). There is always the possibility that they might turn out to be right. But while many of the authors raise valid points in an emotional appeal, unfortunately their credibility often suffers due to the routine use of half-truths, unfounded opinions disguised as facts, and occasional outright falsehoods.

This is not surprising, since virtually all of them are unfamiliar with production agriculture, biology, and genetics. Still, they bring up some important issues for our consideration. But the tendency of these bloggers to play fast and loose with the facts makes it very easy to be suspicious of their integrity and their motives. They may well have good intentions, but do they actually understand the issues? And are they being objective? One of the most troubling problems is the consistent absence of any valid scientific proof to support their claims. Some insist that they have proof, but closer scrutiny invariably reveals that it does not meet the standards of acceptable science.

That certainly doesn't mean that the proof is not out there somewhere, just waiting to be discovered. But it does suggest that with so many people actively searching for some way to provide indisputable scientific proof of adverse effects, if any such proof does indeed exist, it should have been found and widely published by now.

The bottom line is, scientific proof is the only way we have to separate fact from fiction. The caveat about that statement is the observation that even scientifically-proven claims are occasionally proven to be wrong because of corrupt science.

## So we must remain objective.

History proves (with a 99 % extinction rate) that all it takes is one major fault (or more often, a number of smaller ones), and our own species may become a candidate for extinction. We have so many harmful ingredients in so many of our foods, that tracking down the exact cause of any resulting health problem can be a daunting challenge. Who knows . . . proof of adverse effects from GMOs might be found tomorrow — or it might never be found.

## Be that as it may, no one should be forced against their will to accept genetically modified foods for their own consumption.

Today, some non -GMO options are still available. But sadly, in the distant future, those options will probably no longer exist. The report acknowledges that already a few examples can be found where certain GM traits have crossed over to certain related wild species (because of natural cross-breeding). Since the pollen of a GM plant can transfer GM traits to the seeds of a non-GM plant, eventually most (or all) plants will likely possess GM characteristics. In the case of genetic modifications, once the cat is out of the bag, it cannot be put back in — and unfortunately the cat is long since out of the bag, with regard to most existing GM commercial seeds. This is most likely the scariest part of the entire GM issue. It's probably already too late to go back, even if we wanted.

## But then, our ancestors had to deal with basically the same dilemma as the neolithic period unfolded.

Those tribes that chose to continue with a hunter-gatherer way of life should not have been forced to accede to an agricultural lifestyle, either. But the rules of progress don't always allow such choices. We learn to embrace whatever society embraces, or we suffer the consequences. It has always been that way and that is unlikely to change, now or in the future.

Unfortunately the archaeological evidence indicates that the remaining hunter-gatherers didn't actually have much choice. As farming slowly replaced the hunter-gatherer lifestyle in the neolithic period it became a juggernaut and the remaining hunter-gatherer tribes who chose not to switch found themselves in a dilemma similar to that faced by those who oppose GM today. Their fate was described by Jared Diamond as follows (Diamond, 1987):

> *As population densities of hunter-gatherers slowly rose at the end of the ice ages, bands had to choose between feeding more mouths by taking the first steps toward agriculture, or else finding ways to limit growth. Some bands chose the former solution, unable to anticipate the evils of farming, and seduced by the transient abundance they enjoyed until population growth caught up with increased food production. Such bands outbred and then drove off or killed the bands that chose to remain hunter-gatherers, because a hundred malnourished farmers can still outfight one healthy hunter. It's not that hunter-gatherers abandoned their life style, but that those sensible enough not to abandon it were forced out of all areas except the ones farmers didn't want.* (p. 66)

# Chapter 5

# Do Consumers Actually Understand Food Safety Issues?

## The evidence suggests that most consumers may misunderstand many issues concerning food

An unfortunate side effect of the first generations of GMOs has been a huge increase in the use of glyphosate and a few other herbicides that are viewed by some as toxic. And this has been a focus of the general public campaign against the use of GMOs. Clearly, the Monsanto chairman of the board of directors doesn't start each meeting by asking "What can we do to benefit the general health of the public today?" That would be absurd.

Obviously it's much more likely that the primary focus of the board (as always) is "What can we do today to improve our sales and profits?" And that shouldn't be surprising, since that's what the shareholders elected them to do in the first place. That's just good business. But this problem needs to be addressed. Aside from any claimed toxicity, a shift toward the use of massive amounts of any chemical is not a good policy in the long run. How is that progress? GMOs are claimed to be a benefit for everyone, not just farmers. The reality is, this hasn't happened, at least not so far.

It's true that GM procedures have allowed the development of synthetic food products such as meat alternatives (Impossible Burger) and vanilla flavoring made from GM yeast. It has also allowed the development of the "Arctic Apple", which does not turn brown when sliced. But considering what the first two are derived from, and considering that we evolved eating whole, natural foods, are these synthetic foods actually "food"? Conventional apples turn brown after slicing if not eaten promptly. So what? Why is that a problem that must be corrected? In other words, from a practical viewpoint, are these good uses of science?

The Impossible Burger for example is not free of issues. Apparently the "heme" protein that gives it the red meat color may be an allergen. And according to Friends of the Earth, the product contains 46 unassessed proteins, and FDA documents state that the studies submitted by the manufacturer "do not establish the safety" of the product (Perls, 2017, Oct 11).[24] With that many new proteins, what percentage of consumers' immune systems will react adversely? And because of the lack of a legal definition of the term "natural", Evolva is marketing it's yeast-derived vanillin as natural, even though it is a product of a GMO.

Arguably, a primary health problem is caused by the fact that most conventionally grown produce (not just GMOs) contain chemical residues from pesticides. A recently-published Shopper's Guide from the EWG (Environmental Working Group) points out that according to a United States Department of Agriculture (USDA) report, recent tests showed that almost 70 % of the samples tested in 2016 were contaminated with pesticide residues (News Release, 2018, Apr 10).[25] Their guide lists what they refer to as the "Dirty Dozen" (fruits and vegetables that contain the highest levels of pesticide residues), and the Clean Fifteen (produce that contained the lowest levels or no detectable pesticide residues at all).

The guide points out (among other things) that over 98 % of the apples, cherries, nectarines, peaches, potatoes, and strawberries tested showed positive results for one or more pesticides. On the other hand, over 80 % of the asparagus, cabbages, onions, papayas, and pineapples tested showed no pesticide residues. And less than 1 % of the avocados and sweet corn tested showed any residues at all.

While pesticide residues may be a more serious problem than any risks currently imposed by GMOs, they are a separate issue and no one seems to be classifying this risk according to GMO or non-GMO status. Instead of analyzing known problems, everyone seems to have tunnel vision and they are focused on a perceived (but unproven) threat from GMOs.

Aren't we worrying about the wrong issue here? We know that pesticide resides in food are harmful to human health. We only suspect that GMOs are a threat, simply because we don't understand them so we're afraid of them. Yet how many blogs have you seen lately about the risks of pesticide residues in food, compared with the number of blogs focusing on GMOs?

## A lot of confusion and misunderstanding about food exists among consumers.

In part this is due to the efforts of anti-this-or-that advocacy groups who realize that if they can spread doubt or confusion about an issue, they can gain supporters of their cause — whether it's legitimate or not. The federal GMO labeling law that was recently passed was in response to state laws in Vermont, Connecticut, and Maine that were passed because of public distrust of GMO safety.

But a survey taken in 2016 (known as the Annenberg Science Knowledge survey project) discovered that even though 88 % of the respondents supported mandatory labeling laws, 58 % admitted that their understanding of GMOs was either fair or poor (PR Newswire, 2016, Jul 18).[26] And over 80 % were not even aware that scientists have not been able to find any evidence that GMOs have any adverse effects on human health.

While we're on the topic of confusion about food among consumers, it might be a good time to look at consumer beliefs about organic foods. This might help to illustrate the level of misunderstanding among consumers about food issues in general.

## Is organically-produced food actually better than conventionally-produced food?

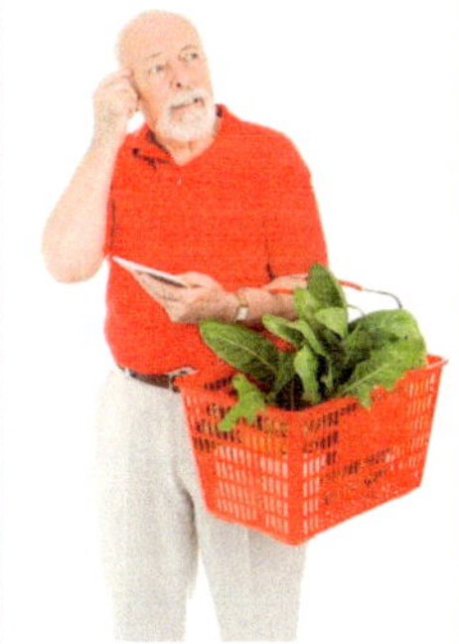

*Illustration 16: Shoppers are often confused by food claims.*

We would like to believe that it is. And most people do believe that it is. But what we would like to believe, and actual fact, are sometimes two different things. Back in December of 2016, a report was released by the research arm of the European Parliament. The report was intended to be based on published scientific evidence associated with the agricultural production of organic food. It was noted that people who eat organic foods are often the same people who have healthier diets to begin with, and this makes it very difficult to attribute their healthy status to the consumption of organic food. Obviously their better health might simply be due to their better diet in general. But the bottom line in the report was that they could not confirm that eating organically produced food offered any proven health benefits. Specifically, they concluded that (GMO FAQ, n.d.):[27]

> *" In conclusion, there is a lack of data from well-designed studies (prospective, long-term duration, accurate data in particular for dietary factors and sources, i.e. conventional or organic) involving a sufficiently large population."*

## The fact that organic foods could not be shown to be superior to conventional foods had been pointed out previously.

In a Scientific American Article called Mythbusting 101, for example, Christie Wilcox had pointed out that (Wilcox, 2011, July 18):[28]

1. Organic farms do indeed use pesticides (only approved types)
2. Organic foods have not been proven to be healthier
3. Organic farming is not better for the environment
4. Organic farming is not an all or none issue

## Similar claims could be made for the "conventional-crops-versus-GMOs" issue.

It could be argued that:

1. Conventional farms use the same chemicals
2. Conventional foods have not been proven to be healthier
3. Conventional farming is not better for the environment
4. Conventional farming is not an all or none issue.

## We believe what we want to believe.

When reading articles about any given topic, research proves that people tend to believe information that is consistent with their own desires and/or beliefs (Bastardi, Uhlmann, & Ross, 2011).[29] And conversely, they are less likely to believe information that conflicts with their own desires or beliefs. In other words, we tend to believe claims about issues (usually without question) when those claims happen to coincide with our own beliefs. And this happens without our realization that our own desires are influencing our perception of the evidence. Obviously, this makes the job of changing someone's opinion much more difficult after they've formed an initial opinion.

# Chapter 6

# The Future of GM

## What could happen next?

To provide the potential benefits associated with GM, the technology must overcome current public fears. As long as there is fear, there will be distrust. Surely the scientific community is smart enough to be able to erase the fears by replacing them with transparency and understanding.

That said, it's difficult to ignore the most significant problem with the entire program. A decade ago we thought that GM methods would lead to foods that taste better and have longer shelf lives. We thought that the technology would bring us more nutritious foods and even foods that help to fight diseases, including foods that fight cancer (Ardent Editor, 2007, Feb 23).[30] While some of those things have happened, the improvements haven't generally been overly impressive.

Development of a GMO typically requires many years (decades), but we will almost surely eventually see disease-resistant pigs and chickens that are immune to bird flu, for example. Drought-resistant, higher-yielding crops will surely be coming, also. And new treatment methods for cancer and many other diseases will eventually be created.

There is even talk of bringing back from extinction certain organisms that disappeared from the earth long ago. Woolly mammoths survived until about 4,000 years ago. We may have enough DNA from them, and certain other plants and animals, that we will be able to resurrect them.

But more than just a technology issue, this is an ethical issue, and opinions vary widely on just how far scientists should be allowed to go. In view of the fact that we seem to feel that no expense should be spared (especially as long as it's somebody else's money) in attempting to prevent the extinction of virtually any organism alive today (that's facing extinction), shouldn't we be eager to bring back creatures that are already extinct? That would be an even better use of our resources. Or would it?

"Un-extincting" organisms would invalidate Darwin's theory of evolution (because extinction is an integral part of evolution, according to the theory). And it would presumably ignore various other laws of nature and the universe, for that matter. But some day (assuming our continuing tenure on this planet) we will have to make that decision.

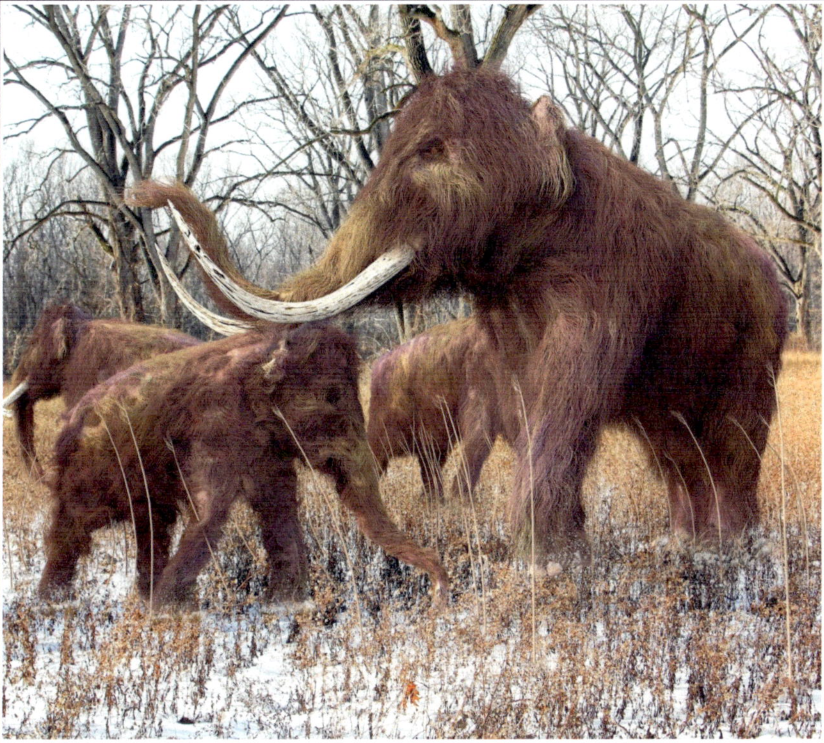

*Illustration 17: Woolly mammoth family — are we capable of bring them back from extinction? Should we try?*

## There are a lot of questions about which way future developments may proceed.

While the U.S. Government's position on GMOs seems to be "full steam ahead as long as you follow the regulations", the EU continues to block GMO research. They allow individual countries to decide for themselves whether they will allow the importation of GMO products while banning research on, and growing

GMO crops. The primary obstacle appears to be their broad definition of GMO.

Europe generated their regulations (Directive 1829/2003) on GM crops in the 1990s and early 2000s and adopted them in 2004. But the directive defines a GMO as "an organism in which the genetic material has been altered in a way that does not occur naturally" (Nigel Halford, 2018, Mar 14).[31] Obviously this definition is so broad that it even applies to many conventionally-used plant breeding techniques (in addition to GM processes). So biotechnology is severely compromised in Europe and biotech companies have abandoned trying to develop new crops there.

## Beyond GM technology lies the development of what's known as synthetic biology.

GM methods normally involve the removal or addition of just one or two individual genes. Synthetic biology (or synbio for short) involves the creation of organisms with not just one or two new genes, but clusters of new genes.

But an early and highly-visible attempt to demonstrate to doubters just how great synthetic biology could be, failed miserably. And the venture (known as the glowing plant project), which was funded by almost half-a-million dollars from hopeful supporters on Kickstarter, was declared officially "dead" after about four years of fruitless work. The initial idea was to create a glowing Arabidopsis thaliana plant and then to move on to developing trees that would glow and replace street lamps. But the first step required the insertion of six genes at one time, and the research team soon discovered that this was much easier said than done. They did manage to get a little glow (enough to be faintly seen in the dark), but not enough to matter. The project leader finally had to "pull the plug" when the project ran out of money, without any significant progress to show for all the time and money that had been invested.

It's interesting to note that this project did not fall under any regulatory authority, since it was located within the borders of the United States. It was exempt from FDA and USDA regulation because it was not a food or pharmaceutical item and so it wasn't covered by their guidelines. And since it didn't pose a risk to existing native plants, the Animal and Plant Health Inspection Service (APHIS) had no reason to be interested. But the project would not have been legal in Europe because of stricter EU rules that prohibit such research.

In addition to some unhappy supporters, part of the fallout from this project was a change in policy at Kickstarter. Synthetic biology projects are no longer allowed by the website.

## As GMOs become more complex, risk assessment will almost surely become more difficult.

Guidelines at regulatory agencies will need to be updated to cover new, increasingly-complex technology that might or might not impose new threats to the environment, or to human or animal health. Regulators will have to design ways to eliminate the possibility that unforeseen risks might slip through the cracks.

## Look at how far we've come.

About 10,000 years ago our species was facing the grim specter of starvation. By applying biotechnology to a couple of lucky events in nature (the hybridization of wheat), today we have such robust food security that even with the reality of a continually-expanding global population, we believe we have earned the luxury of choosing to decline new technology. But as we saw in chapter 3, we have always felt that way. History will prove whether we actually have that option.

In our past, despite objections to virtually every technological advancement that has ever come along, technology has always prevailed. And we have always benefited from it in one way or another.

## What will happen if we not only do not benefit from new technology, but suffer some type of severe damage instead?

Or what will happen if new technological developments do not prevail? Will we once again be facing the possibility of starvation a few generations down the road? Regardless of our chosen course of action, the future is always an unknown, and humans always fear the unknown. So clearly, the future is likely to be concerning. But looking back on our track record, we will surely adjust and move on. If there is one virtue of our species that can be pointed to as the reason why we have evolved to our current status, its the fact that humans are very, very adaptable, whether they are willing to admit it or not.

# About the Author

## Wayne Persky BSME

Wayne Persky was born, grew up, and currently lives in Central Texas. He is a graduate of the University of Texas at Austin, College of Engineering, with postgraduate studies in mechanical engineering, mathematics, and computer science. He has teaching experience in engineering, and business experience in farming and agribusiness.

After the onset of severe digestive system and general health problems in the late 1990s, he went through extensive clinical testing, but the GI specialist failed to take biopsies during a colonoscopy exam, and even failed to test for celiac disease. Afterward, not surprisingly, he was told by his gastroenterologist that there was nothing wrong with him.

Unable to find a medical solution, he was forced to use his research skills to discover innovative ways to resolve his health issues. After extensive study, he identified the likely source of the problem as food sensitivities.

It took a year and a half of avoiding all traces of gluten, plus trial and error experimentation with other foods, and careful record-keeping, to track down all of the food issues. But once he eliminated all of them from his diet, he got his life back. He currently administrates an online microscopic colitis discussion and support forum, while continuing to live on a farm in Central

Texas. In 2015 he founded the Microscopic Colitis Foundation and he continues to serve as president and as a contributing author to the Newsletter.

# Contact Details:

Wayne Persky can be contacted at:
Persky Farms
19242 Darrs Creek Rd
Bartlett, TX 76511
USA

Tel: 1(254)718-1125
Tel: 1(254)527-3682

Email: wayne@perskyfarms.com
Email: wayne@microscopiccolitisfoundation.org
Email: wayne@waynepersky.com

My author website can be found at http://www.waynepersky.com/

1 Why is the Wheat Genome So Complicated? (2013, November 15). Colorado Wheat. Retrieved from http://coloradowheat.org/2013/11/why-is-the-wheat-genome-so-complicated/

2 Triticum dicoccon. (n.d.). *Encyclopedia of Life*. Retrieved from http://eol.org/pages/1114086/overview

3 Triticum monococcum. (n.d.). *Encyclopedia of Life*. Retrieved from http://eol.org/pages/1115242/overview

4 Crop Origins. (n.d.). Chelsea Flower Show. Retrieved from https://www.jic.ac.uk/chelsea/crop_origins.htm

5 Triticum aestivum. (n.d). *Encyclopedia of Life*. Retrieved from http://eol.org/pages/1115240/details

6 Tye-Din, J. A., Stewart, J. A., Dromey, J. A., Beissbarth, T., van Heel, D. A., Tatham, A., . . . Anderson, R. P. (2010). Comprehensive, quantitative mapping of T cell epitopes in gluten in celiac disease. Science Translational Medicine, 2(41), 41–51. Retrieved from https://www.ncbi.nlm.nih.gov/pubmed/20650871

7 Guandalini, S. (2007, summer). A brief history of celiac disease. *Impact, The University of Chicago Celiac Disease Center.* 7(3). Retrieved from https://www.cureceliacdisease.org/wp-content/uploads/SU07CeliacCtr.News_.pdf

8 National Academies of Sciences, Engineering, and Medicine; Health and Medicine Division; Food and Nutrition Board; Committee on Food Allergies: Global Burden, Causes, Treatment, Prevention, and Public Policy; Stallings, V. A., & Oria,

M. P. (Eds). (2017). *Finding a path to safety in food allergy: Assessment of the global burden, causes, prevention, management, and public policy.* Washington, D.C.: The National Academies of Sciences, Engineering, & Medicine, Retrieved from https://www.nap.edu/catalog/23658/finding-a-path-to-safety-in-food-allergy-assessment-of

9 Wanjek, C. (2012, Movember 26). Sorry, vegans: Eating meat and cooking food is how humans got their big brains. *The Washington Post: Health and Science,* Retrieved from http://www.washingtonpost.com/national/health-science/sorry-vegans-eating-meat-and-cooking-food-is-how-humans-got-their-big-brains/2012/11/26/3d4d36de-326d-11e2-bb9b-288a310849ee_story.html

10 Choi, C. Q. (2012, October 3). Eating meat made us human, suggests new skull fossil. Live Science, Retrieved from https://www.livescience.com/23671-eating-meat-made-us-human.html

11 Choi, C. Q. (2011, December 13). Bulging brain structures separate us from neanderthals. Live Science, Retrieved from https://www.livescience.com/17441-neanderthal-brains-modern-humans.html

12 Lund University. (2018, March 19). Fish accounted for surprisingly large part of the Stone Age diet. Retrieved from https://www.sciencedaily.com/releases/2018/03/180319120536.htm

13 Diamond, J. (1999, May 01). From the May, 1987 issue of Discover magazine. *The worst mistake in the history of the human race.* Retrieved from http://discovermagazine.com/1987/may/02-the-worst-mistake-in-the-history-of-the-human-race

14 AP. (1988, July 20). Farm population lowest since 1850's. p. A00012. Retrieved from https://www.nytimes.com/1988/07/20/us/farm-population-lowest-since-1850-s.html

15 Halweil, B. (2000, September). Where Have All the Farmers Gone? World Watch Magazine, 13, (5). Retrieved from http://www.worldwatch.org/node/490

16 Ball, P. (2010, May 24). "Playing God" is a meaningless, dangerous cliché. *Prospect Magazine,* Retrieved from https://www.prospectmagazine.co.uk/science-and-technology/playing-god-is-a-meaningless-dangerous-cliche

17 Technology Spotlight. (2017, Feb 1). The science inside a GMO seed. Retrieved from https://modernag.org/innovation/the-science-inside-gmo-seeds/?gclid=EAIaIQobChMIoYuRp6Tn2-gIVgp6fCh3YNACqEAMYASAAEgJxjPD_BwE&gclsrc=aw.ds

18 Raymond, M. and Kubitz, L. (2016, May 11). *Survey: Food Dialogue Gains Momentum; Media Drive Beliefs, Changes.* Retrieved from http://www.foodinsight.org/press-releases/survey-food-dialogue-gains-momentum-media-drive-beliefs-changes

19 Nature Education. (2014). Genetically modified organisms (GMOs). Retrieved from https://www.nature.com/scitable/spotlight/gmos-6978241#spArticleViewHdr

20 The Times Editorial Board. (2016, May 21). Moving beyond the GMO "Frankenfood" debate. Los Angeles Times, Retrieved from http://www.latimes.com/opinion/editorials/la-ed-gmo-report-20160522-snap-story.html

21 News Release. (2016, May 17). Distinction between genetic engineering and conventional plant breeding becoming less clear, says new report on GE crops. *National Academies of Sciences, Engineering, and Medicine,* Retrieved from http://www8.nationalacademies.org/onpinews/newsitem.aspx?RecordID=23395

22 U. S. Department of Health & Human Sevices: National Institutes of Health: U. S. National Library of Medicine. (2018). *What are genome editing and CRISPR-Cas9?* Retrieved from https://ghr.nlm.nih.gov/primer/genomicresearch/genomeediting

23 debating europe. (n.d.). Arguments for and against GMOs. Retrieved from http://www.debatingeurope.eu/focus/arguments-gmos/#.Wu5arztG2mx

24 Dana Perls. (2017, Oct 11). The future of food: The next generation of GMOs. Friends of the Earth, Retrieved from https://foe.org/future-food-next-generation-gmos/

25 News Release. (2018, Apr 10). Out Now: EWG's 2018 Shopper's Guide to pesticides in produce™. Environmental Working Group, Retrieved from https://www.ewg.org/release/out-now-ewg-s-2018-shopper-s-guide-pesticides-produce#.Wu8xtjtG2mz

26 PR Newswire. (2016, Jul 18). Americans support GMO food labels but don't know much about safety of genetically modified foods. The Annenberg Public Policy Center of the University of Pennsylvania, Retrieved from https://www.prnewswire.com/news-releases/americans-support-gmo-food-labels-but-dont-know-much-about-safety-of-genetically-modified-foods-300300115.html

27 GMO FAQ. (n.d.). Are organic foods healthier than conventional foods? Retrieved from https://gmo.geneticliteracyproject.org/FAQ/are-organic-foods-healthier-than-conventional-foods/

28 Christie Wilcox. (2011, July 18). Mythbusting 101: Organic farming > Conventional agriculture. Retrieved from https://blogs.scientificamerican.com/science-sushi/httpblogsscientificamericancomscience-sushi20110718mythbusting-101-organic-farming-conventional-agriculture/

29 Bastardi, A., Uhlmann, W. L., & Ross, L. (2011). Wishful thinking: Belief, desire,and the motivated evaluation of scientific evidence. Psychological Science, 22(6), 731–732. Retrieved from http://journals.sagepub.com/doi/full/10.1177/0956797611406447

30 Ardent Editor. (2007, Feb 23). The future of genetically modified (GM) foods. Genetic Modifications, Retrieved from http://gm.org/2007/02/23/the-future-of-genetically-modified-gm-foods/

31 Nigel Halford. (2018, Mar 14). Europe missed out on GMO biotech revolution. What's going to happen with gene editing? Retrieved from https://geneticliteracyproject.org/2018/03/14/europe-missed-out-on-gmo-biotech-revolution-whats-going-to-happen-with-gene-editing/

Made in United States
Cleveland, OH
05 November 2026

47664330R00048